A GUIDE TO PHYSICAL THERAPY FOR HORSES

A Guide to Physical Training and Therapeutic Aids of Horses

Lincoln Betty

Table of Contents

CHAPTER I

Preface

Physiotherapy entails assessing the capability of the body to move and perform bodily interest. It consists of searching at joint mobility, muscle length and energy, coordination, stability and the ability to perform sure responsibilities. The physiotherapist's aims are to reduce pain and swelling and enhance movement and characteristic of the patient. They use some of one of a kind strategies, such as massage, warm and cold remedies, hydrotherapy, laser, myofascial launch, joint mobilizations and acupuncture, and use sports to increase variety of motion, support muscle mass and enhance stability and coordination.

How healing exercise applications can help maintain equine athletes and leisure horses alike feeling their quality

Physical remedy. When you pay attention those phrases, you would possibly reflect in consideration on regular office visits for supervised stretches, sports, and icing, all inside the name of rehabbing from damage or easing aches and pains.

But bodily therapy can follow to horses, too. Physical therapists like me work with horses to help them optimize motion, get over injuries, and attain height performance. In this text we'll speak the fundamentals of equine physical therapy and the way it might assist your horse.

CHAPTER II

The Four Pinnacles of Equine Physical Therapy

Trained and authorized bodily therapists use a complete assessment model addressing 4 key regions to assist equine athletes stay sound or recover from damage. After veterinary diagnosis and referral of the case, therapists start by determining if horses have complete range of motion. Second, they verify whether sufferers can pass thru that full variety. If now not, the animals are maximum likely lame—and the veterinarian desires to live worried.

The 0.33 vicinity therapists examine and manipulate is motor manage, which entails assessing and retraining dynamic power and stability. For instance, a horse with poor core electricity may warfare to carry out a canter transition without throwing his head within the air. Identifying that core electricity is proscribing his ability to push into the canter is an example of addressing the problem, no longer a symptom. In this situation, core strengthening physical games, consisting of lateral tail pulls or walking over extended cavalettis, might be more effective than practicing canter transitions time and again.

The fourth vicinity to assess and optimize is the pony's capacity to deal with load. This consists of sporting a rider and possessing the energy and motor manage to carry out more superior actions, along with leaping fences or changing leads.

One of the best tools to retrain and enhance these regions is a therapeutic exercising software. Therapists design these applications to improve the movement deficits they identified at the evaluation. They alter and improve them through the years to assist the horse development, return to his previous level of performance, or attain peak performance

CHAPTER III

Which Horses Need Physiotherapy?

Physiotherapy can assist to alleviate aches, ache and stiffness associated with arthritis (degenerative joint sickness) and the getting older technique. Many horses develop degenerative joint disorder early in existence because of increase costs, congenital troubles, previous damage and from time to time the nature of the work they perform.

• Stretching

• Back, neck and sacroiliac ache

- Tendon and muscle harm

- Arthritis

- Exercise and Performance

- Nerve injuries

- Rehabilitation after harm or surgical operation

- **The Injured Horse**

The horse is an elite athlete, and need to accept the hazard to reach the most beneficial stage of overall performance. Physiotherapy helps to reap and maintain performance inside the equine athlete.

Horses broaden again and neck pain and different musculoskeletal injuries due to the nature in their paintings. Specific musculoskeletal injuries consist of tendon and smooth tissue injuries from everyday work and overtraining, as well as pressure fractures, fractures and nerve accidents, from falls and accidents.

Following preliminary veterinary prognosis, in the acute segment of injury, physiotherapy enables to lessen pain, swelling and inflammation, and starts to restore the pony's motion. Physiotherapists can then offer full and ongoing rehabilitation to purpose to repair the equine athlete's overall performance.

- **Back Pain**

Back, neck and sacroiliac ache are not unusual inside the overall performance and leisure horse. The physiotherapists use manipulation, and other spinal mobilization strategies to repair motion and decrease ache bobbing up from the vertebral column and sacroiliac joint within the horse. Exercises are typically prescribed, to help hold the feature within the backbone.

- **After Surgery**

Physiotherapy intervention following equine arthroscopic joint surgical procedure, surgical restore of tendons and fractures, and belly surgical treatment (together with colic) can enhance the pony's recuperation. The accurate rehabilitation guarantees most excellent return to characteristic.

- **Prevention of Injury**

Early detection of motion abnormalities, which may be

Indicative of orthopedic situations, muscle imbalances or other musculoskeletal issues, is important to assist prevent development or worsening of ache and lack of overall performance.

The physiotherapists are well certified to evaluate motion disorders, and speak closely with veterinarians who will diagnose if there is an underlying condition.

- **The Aged Horse And Arthritic Joints**

Physiotherapy can assist to relieve aches, ache and stiffness related to arthritis (degenerative joint ailment) and the growing older method. Many horses broaden degenerative joint ailment early in lifestyles because of increase prices, congenital issues, preceding harm and now and again the nature of the work they perform. Performance horses can still remain aggressive with arthritic adjustments, presenting they are controlled with veterinary care and with physiotherapy. Physiotherapy can help to prolong a horse's years of activity, or without a doubt offer a higher exceptional of lifestyles.

- **Competition Horses**

These horses will be placing a whole lot of stress on their frame due to the excessive intensity paintings that they're doing. Especially if they may be at a high degree of opposition. Just like a human athlete, regular physiotherapy ought to be carried out to make sure that they're in height physical health; it is able to assist enhance overall performance, save you harm, and beautify mobility and flexibility, being essential not only during top education, however additionally in the course of rest and recovery periods.

- **Routine Test-Ups**

It's no longer best the elite athletes that want physiotherapy. Carrying out a habitual evaluation is on occasion endorsed for all horses, assisting to come across small troubles early. Ensuring that your horse is ache unfastened and has an awesome variety of movement is important to allow them to stay a satisfied and healthy existence, enabling them to do the paintings this is required of them. In maximum cases a routine physiotherapy evaluation is recommended every 6-twelve months. However, in case your horse has a records of musculoskeletal issues, they may require greater common test-ups.

- **Horses Which Are Rehabilitating After Musculoskeletal Accidents**

Following damage or surgical operation, physiotherapy is crucial to help to lessen irritation, enhance strength and growth variety of movement, with the aim of restoring the animal again to full characteristic. Soft tissue techniques can be used to loosen up scars, swollen joints and thickened tissues after injury. A strict exercise regime will normally be created to encourage the perfect use of the affected region.

CHAPTER IV

How Do You Know If Your Horse Wishes a Physiotherapy Assessment

As nicely as getting an ordinary test-up via the physiotherapist, your horse may also want to see them on different occasions. Any adjustments to the manner your horse is acting may additionally need assessment through a physiotherapist as those may want to suggest symptoms of musculoskeletal ache. Signs consist of anxiety via the neck and lower back when placing the saddle on, reluctance to jump or canter on one rein, stiffness on one aspect or bucking. The symptoms may additionally even be extra subtle, together with facial modifications, uneven shoe wear or changes in ear position while using. At first, it may seem like the pony is being naughty however it is vital to have your horse checked over as all of those symptoms could be associated with nark, returned or pelvic pain. Ensuring which you watch your horse intently is vital to be able to pick up any troubles quickly.

What's an Exercise Program?

Therapeutic exercising is designed to clear up a selected hassle, consisting of stifle weak spot or loss of center muscle engagement. The purpose is to help your horse pass optimally and take care of the demands of his sport and workload. A comprehensive healing exercise application addresses:

• Range of movement Do the pony's joints have full range of movement?

• Proprioception Does your horse know where his frame is in

area? You frequently must retrain this system after an injury and/or if your horse has been in ache.

• Motor manage how does your horse regulate how he starts off evolved, movements via, and ends a motion?

• Strength Does your horse have adequate power for his job?

• Endurance Can your horse produce enough power to perform?

• Speed Can your horse competently circulate rapid sufficient for the needs of the game?

A top exercising application addresses a majority of these areas and focuses on innovative overload—applying strain to the gadget in small, prepared increments to create physiological diversifications inclusive of increasing muscular tissues, building more blood vessels, strengthening connective tissue, and increasing nerve conduction velocity.

Conditioned sufferers tend to get injured much less regularly than the below- or over conditioned ones. "I regularly see humans competing on a horse that isn't fit or riding the horse beyond the point of fatigue, and I experience this is where a massive percentage of accidents arise," he says. "There are continually going to be the fluke injuries that cannot be avoided; however, once a horse is tired, that horse can no longer protect his body."

Therapeutic Training Aids

A type of training equipment can assist enhance a horse's range of movement, frame cognizance, neurologic integration, and energy. Work with your veterinarian or bodily therapist to determine which schooling aids to consist of for your software. Remember, those gear are handiest as excellent as the exercising software your vet or therapist prescribes to your horse and the ability of the rider or trainer the usage of them. It's crucial to know the cause behind the use of a training resource and incorporating it into a remedy plan, as opposed to just arbitrarily adding it into the mix.

Tactile Bracelets

These light-weight bracelets may be located on the pony's pasterns to stimulate the pores and skin and growth the flight arc of the leg (Clayton et al., 2008). They educate the horse to lift a foot better off the floor—beneficial if he drags a toe or doesn't elevate a previously injured leg as high as the noninjured one. The primary issue with these bracelets is horses can get desensitized speedy. Think approximately how you could wear a watch and neglect you have got it on. The bracelets will have the equal effect but are beneficial for quick sessions.

Used for: Range of movement

Leg Weights

Like tactile bracelets, including a small amount of weight to a horse's leg can reason the horse to stroll with an exaggerated stepping motion due to the fact he must contract extra proximal (closer to the frame/factor of attachment) muscle groups to lift the heavier leg. In my practice I actually have used this method to build stifle power after an damage. Excessive weight or overuse, but, can injure tender tissues.

Used for: Range of motion, proprioception, electricity

Foam Pads and Wedges

Commercial foam pads are useful for enhancing range of movement and proprioception. The horse stands on the pads, which demanding situations the postural muscle mass and proprioceptive device. Some pads also come in wedge shape, which could assist increase variety of motion by lightly stretching connective tissues within the lower limbs.

Used for: Range of movement, proprioception, electricity

Resistance Band Structures

These gear boom core and spinal muscle activation. Researchers (Pfau et al., 2017) have proven band systems assist growth thoracolumbar balance and decrease the chance of pain or injury from hollowing the returned.

Used for: Strength, proprioception

Ground Poles

Poles are one of the most beneficial gear to assist enhance decrease limb variety of movement, strength, and proprioception. You can area them at the ground or increase them up to 8 inches and have your horse stroll or trot over them. You also can region poles in an prepared sample, which includes 3 to 4 ft apart, or scattered randomly so the pony have to navigate his way via a maze. Small soar fences also are extremely useful to enhance response time and power.

Used for: Range of movement, proprioception, strength, velocity

Aquatic Treadmills

These motive a horse to walk with extended joint flexion and lift his legs better off the floor. They also can help construct strength and patience as the pony pulls in opposition to the water. Depending on the water depth, the pony would possibly experience a buoyancy effect that reduces impact at the leg joints, which is beneficial for the duration of restoration from accidents inclusive of tendon or ligament traces.

Used for: Range of motion, electricity, staying power

THE END